first place
4health

food on the go
pocket guide

Published by Gospel Light
Ventura, California, U.S.A.
www.gospellight.com
Printed in the U.S.A.

All information contained in the tables
of this guide are accurate as of March 2008.

Rights for publishing this book outside the U.S.A.
or in non-English languages are administered by
Gospel Light Worldwide, an international not-for-profit
ministry. For additional information, please visit
www.glww.org, email info@glww.org, or write
to Gospel Light Worldwide, 1957 Eastman Avenue,
Ventura, CA 93003, U.S.A.

contents

RESTAURANT GUIDE

about
first place 4 health

Seek first his kingdom and his righteousness,
and all these things will be given to you as well.

MATTHEW 6:33

The First Place 4 Health program was developed more than 25 years ago out of a godly desire placed in the hearts of a group of Christians to establish a Christ-centered weight-control program. Since then, it has evolved into a nationally recognized total-health program.

First Place 4 Health addresses all areas of a person's life—spiritual, mental, emotional and physical—through Bible study, small-group support, accountability, a commonsense nutrition plan, exercise, record-keeping and Scripture memory. It is used by people in every U.S. state and many foreign countries. Thousands of lives have been changed!

eating healthy
when eating out

National survey data shows a significant trend in the dining styles of most Americans over the past few decades: Eating away from home is increasing in popularity. The number of people who ate out one or more meal per week and those who ate out three or more meals per week was 40 percent higher in 2000 than in 1987.[1] Whether for time and convenience, variety or value, Americans waste no time pulling into the local drive-thru or diner—even for breakfast!

Unfortunately, higher eating-out frequency is associated with adverse nutritional consequences. Although many consumers agree that they are responsible for making their own sensible food choices away from home, French fries continue to trump green salads as the more popular choice for a side dish.

Believe it or not, you can dine out without blowing it—you just need to know how! The keys to success are (1) making a plan for healthy eating, (2) sticking with it, and (3) asking for exactly what you want.

You've got to fight for your right to eat healthy! When you breeze through the doors of your favorite restaurant, you are not entering a new world where calories don't count and fat doesn't exist. Rather, calories can add up even quicker and fat is usually lurking around every corner. It is your responsibility to overcome the temptation to let ignorance be your bliss. (And to remind yourself that the bliss will come to a screeching halt the next morning when you try to button your pants.)

The First Place 4 Health *Food on the Go Pocket Guide* will help you as you make your plan. Let's get started!

Note
 1. A. K. Kant and B. I. Graubard, "Eating Out in America, 1987–2000: Trends and Nutritional Correlates," *Preventive Medicine* issue 38 (2004), pp. 243-249.

how to use the
food on the go pocket guide

The First Place 4 Health *Food on the Go Pocket Guide* provides nutrition information about hundreds of menu items found at more than 40 of North America's most popular restaurants, listed in alphabetical order. Along the top of each page are guides to various nutrition facts about each menu item. Definitions for each column listing are found below.

Calories

Make them count! Look at the number of calories and compare them with the nutrients they offer. Get the biggest nutritional bang not only for your buck but also for your calories. Choosing *nutrient*-dense foods as opposed to *calorie*-dense items will not only help you monitor your weight but also ensure that you get what your body really needs:

proper nutrition! Calories from fat are indicated by the *number* of calories from fat, not the percentage. To determine the percentage, divide the number of calories from fat by the number of total calories. On average, choose more foods with 35 percent or less of the total calories from fat. Not every food you eat has to be less than 35 percent fat—just the overall balance of foods you eat!

Total Fat

Total fat is provided in grams. Based on your calorie goals, monitor your fat intake by total fat grams or by percentage of total calories. Twenty to 35 percent of your diet should come from healthy fats like mono- and polyunsaturated fats and oils such as fish, vegetable oils, nuts and seeds. For example, a person who eats 1,800 calories with a total fat intake of 25 percent would consume approximately 450 calories from fat or 50 grams of fat per day.

Saturated Fat

Knowing the breakdown of fat in a food is just as important as knowing the total amount. Saturated fat is one of the worst things for your health. Compare the labels on similar foods and try to choose foods that have 5 percent daily value (% DV) or less of saturated fat. The American Heart Association (AHA) recommends that saturated fat make up 7 percent or less of your total calories. For a person on a 1,600 calorie (kcal) diet, that equals 112 kcals (1,600 kcals x 0.07) or 12.4 grams of saturated fat per day (112 kcals/9). Those grams of saturated fat can add up really fast if you're not careful!

Trans Fat

Thankfully, trans fat has really been making the headlines lately. All the publicity will hopefully lead to reduced intake of this LDL-raising, HDL-lowering, atherosclerosis-promoting fat in the near future! As much as possible, avoid trans fats by choosing foods with 0 grams trans fat and foods made without hydrogenated or partially hydrogenated oils.

Cholesterol

This is another item to keep as low as possible. Your liver makes enough cholesterol on its own that you really don't need much from your diet at all. The current adult recommendation for dietary cholesterol is no more than 300 mg per day. (Fat content is not necessarily a good measurement of cholesterol content. For example, liver and other organ meats are low in fat but very high in cholesterol.)

Sodium

Salt (sodium chloride or NaCl) contains sodium (Na). High sodium intake is linked to higher blood pressure and hypertension. In 2004, the National Academy of Sciences Institute of Medicine came out with a new dietary reference intake (DRI) for sodium that differs from some food labels. Adults are recommended to aim for only 1,200 to 1,500 mg of sodium per day, with a tolerable upper limit (UL) of 2,300 mg (opposed to the previous UL of 2,400 mg). Intakes over the UL are considered to be harmful to your health. Keep in mind that 2,300 mg of sodium is equal to about only 1 teaspoon of salt! Shocking, isn't it? Most Americans consume closer to 3 teaspoons of salt per day—triple the amount recommended!

Fiber

The goal for adult fiber intake is 21 to 38 grams, depending on age. With so many yummy foods to choose from—rich in whole grains, fruits and vegetables—you can achieve that goal painlessly . . . but you better get started! Fiber lowers cholesterol, fills you up, and keeps your gut happy and running smoothly.

Carbohydrate

The U.S. Dietary Guidelines suggest that most of your calories come from fiber- and antioxidant-rich carbohydrates, then healthy fats, and then lean protein. Carbohydrate-rich foods include fruits, vegetables and grain products like bread, pasta or rice. (Protein-rich foods include meat, poultry, fish, eggs and vegetarian sources such as dried beans and peas, nuts and seeds.) One important thing to keep in mind is that naturally occurring sugars in some foods, such as dairy and fruits, are included in the total grams of carboydrate listed for a product. Thus, a food seemingly high in carbohydrate may actually contain few added sugars (added during processing and preparation). *Added* sugars are the ones to avoid, as they provide more calories without the benefit of added nutrients. So, read ingreadient lists when available and choose foods you know to have less added sugars such as sugar-free products or products sweetened naturally.

Protein

Most Americans get more than enough protein from the foods they eat. You should aim for protein to make up 10 to 15 percent of your total calories. For someone on a 1,600 calorie diet, this would mean that their daily protein intake should be around 40 to 60 grams ([1,600 kcals x 0.10 - 0.15]/4). If you are a vegetarian or a vegan, achieving an adequate protein intake is completely attainable by eating a variety of plant-based, protein-rich foods. Note the grams of protein listed for various items and keep track of your intake with your Live It Tracker if you are concerned about not getting enough—or perhaps too much—protein.

healthy tips
for eating out

Some restaurants do a great job of informing their patrons about the nutritional content of their menu items, but most won't do so unless you ask. The good news is that if they want your business, they will most certainly oblige! So remind yourself that you are paying for not only the experience of the meal but also the meal itself. Get what you paid for—namely, a healthy and delicious product! Don't worry; you're not being picky, you're being *proactive*. So ask questions and act accordingly—it's perfectly polite!

Ask If the Restaurant Will:

- Serve your salad dressing and other condiments on the side
- Substitute fried sides for fresh salad greens or grilled veggies

- Serve margarine rather than butter
- Serve fat-free or low-fat milk rather than whole milk or cream
- Accommodate special requests for menu items
- Bring a side of lemon or lime slices to flavor up your water
- Use whole wheat bread or pasta
- Use less oil when cooking
- Hold the salt or use salt-free seasoning
- Trim visible fat from poultry or meat
- Leave off the sauce or substitute for a different kind
- Split the entrée and bring it out on two separate plates

Choose What Is Better (and Still Very Delicious!)

- Don't waste your calories on sugar-filled beverages with no nutritional value! Opt for water (add some lemon or lime if you wish), unsweetened tea that you can sweeten yourself, fat-free or low-fat milk, or *occasional* diet drinks.
- Start off right with a salad to help you control hunger and feel satisfied sooner. It's also an easy way to get your veggies!
- Order pasta dishes with tomato sauce (marinara) instead of cream-based sauces

(alfredo). Stick to items without creamy sauces or gravies.

- Add little or no butter to your food. If you get out of the habit, you'll likely realize you don't miss anything but the extra calories!
- Bypass the all-you-can-eat buffets and order an item from the menu.
- If chips or bread are served as complimentary appetizers, ask the waiter to bring only one basket and spare yourself the temptation.
- Choose fruit-based desserts most often. Split the rich ones with your companions.

Dare to Compare

Menus are full of food clues if you know what to look for. Start choosing more items cooked using healthier methods. Here's a list of terms to look for:

- Choose most often:
  - Baked
  - Broiled
  - Roasted
  - Braised
  - Poached
  - Steamed
  - Stir-fried
  - Grilled

- Sautéed (with broth, cooking spray or minimal oil)
- Tomato sauce

■ Choose seldom:
  - Deep-fried
  - Pan-fried
  - Sautéed (using a lot of butter or oil)
  - Prime
  - Casserole
  - Breaded
  - Alfredo or cream sauce

Take a Taste Adventure

Maintaining variety in your diet is not only essential for nutrition, but it also makes eating fun and exciting! Experiencing new cuisines from around the world is a wonderful way to earn respect for other cultures as well as tickle your taste buds with fresh and delicious new foods. Many ethnic cuisines offer lots of low-fat, low-calorie choices. Here's a sample of healthy food choices and terms to look for when making your selection:

■ Asian:
  - Jum (poached)
  - Kow (roasted)

- Shu (barbecued)
- Steamed dumplings, rice, chicken or shrimp
- Dishes without MSG

■ Italian
- Red sauces (marinara, pomodoro)
- Primavera (no cream)
- Piccata (lemon)
- Sun-dried tomatoes
- Crushed tomatoes
- Lightly sautéed
- Whole wheat pizza crust

Prepare to Enjoy!

When eating out with family and friends, tell them in advance that you plan to eat healthy. Order what you know is best for you, and don't allow yourself to be tempted by others (including the wait staff!). Also, if you know a meal will be high in calories and fat, choose healthier foods the rest of the day and be sure to be physically active.

restaurant guide

Product	Total Calories	Total Calories from Fat	Total Fat (gm)	Saturated Fat (gm)	Trans Fat (gm)	Cholesterol (mg)	Dietary Fiber (gm)	Sodium (mg)	Carbohydrate (gm)	Protein (gm)

A&W ®

www.awrestaurants.com

Product	Total Calories	Total Calories from Fat	Total Fat (gm)	Saturated Fat (gm)	Trans Fat (gm)	Cholesterol (mg)	Dietary Fiber (gm)	Sodium (mg)	Carbohydrate (gm)	Protein (gm)
Coney Chili Dog	310	160	18	7	1	40	2	870	24	13
Grilled Chicken Sandwich	400	117	13	3	1.5	90	2	1050	35	36
Hamburger	430	190	22	7	3.5	55	2	700	37	21
Hot Dog (plain)	280	150	17	6	1	35	1	710	22	11

Arby's ®

www.arbys.com

Product	Total Calories	Total Calories from Fat	Total Fat (gm)	Saturated Fat (gm)	Trans Fat (gm)	Cholesterol (mg)	Dietary Fiber (gm)	Sodium (mg)	Carbohydrate (gm)	Protein (gm)
Arby's Melt Sandwich	302	110	12	4	1	30	2	921	36	16
Arby's Sauce	15	0	0	0	0	0	0	180	4	0
Chicken Bacon and Swiss Grilled Sandwich	461	151	17	4	0	25	2	1333	52	36
Fruit Cup	35	2	0	0	0	0	1	0	9	0
Junior Roast Beef Sandwich	272	92	10	4	0	29	2	740	34	16

Product	Total Calories	Total Calories from Fat	Total Fat (gm)	Saturated Fat (gm)	Trans Fat (gm)	Cholesterol (mg)	Dietary Fiber (gm)	Sodium (mg)	Carbohydrate (gm)	Protein (gm)

Arby's® (cont.)

Product	Total Calories	Total Calories from Fat	Total Fat (gm)	Saturated Fat (gm)	Trans Fat (gm)	Cholesterol (mg)	Dietary Fiber (gm)	Sodium (mg)	Carbohydrate (gm)	Protein (gm)
Light Buttermilk Ranch Dressing	112	57	6	1	<1	1	1	472	13	1
Market Fresh™ Mini Turkey and Cheese Sandwich	244	40	4	1	0	36	2	784	28	19
Martha's Vineyard™ Salad (without dressing or nuts)	277	71	8	4	0	72	4	451	24	26
Medium Roast Beef	415	186	21	9	1	73	2	1379	34	31
Raspberry Vinaigrette	194	123	14	2	0	0	0	387	18	0
Regular Roast Beef Sandwich	320	123	14	5	.5	44	2	953	34	21
Sante Fe Salad™ (with grilled chicken)	283	77	9	4	0	72	6	521	21	29
Sliced Almonds	81	76	8	1	<1	0	1	0	2	4
Super Roast Beef Sandwich	398	174	19	6	.5	45	2	1060	40	21
Swiss Melt	303	111	12	4	1	29	2	919	27	16

Auntie Anne's™   www.auntieannes.com

Product	Total Calories	Total Calories from Fat	Total Fat (gm)	Saturated Fat (gm)	Trans Fat (gm)	Cholesterol (mg)	Dietary Fiber (gm)	Sodium (mg)	Carbohydrate (gm)	Protein (gm)
Original Stix (without butter)	340	10	1	0	0	0	3	900	72	10
Sweet Mustard	60	15	1.5	1	0	40	0	120	8	<1
Whole Wheat Pretzel	370	40	4.5	1.5	0	10	7	1120	72	11

Baja Fresh ®

www.bajafresh.com

Product	Total Calories	Total Calories from Fat	Total Fat (gm)	Saturated Fat (gm)	Trans Fat (gm)	Cholesterol (mg)	Dietary Fiber (gm)	Sodium (mg)	Carbohydrate (gm)	Protein (gm)
Black Beans	360	20	2.5	1	0	5	26	1120	61	23
Chicken Baja Ensalada®	310	60	7	2	0	110	7	1210	18	46
Chicken Bare Burrito	640	60	7	1	0	75	20	2330	97	45
Classic Soft Chicken Taco	230	90	10	4.5	0	35	2	590	20	16
Classic Soft Mahi Mahi Taco	240	90	10	4.5	0	40	2	490	20	17
Fat-free Salsa Verde (3 oz.)	15	0	0	0	0	0	1	370	3	0
Grilled Mahi Mahi Taco	230	80	9	1.5	0	20	4	300	26	12
Original Baja Chicken Taco	210	45	5	1	0	25	2	230	28	12
Pinto Beans	320	10	1	0	0	5	21	840	56	19
Rice	280	35	4	.5	0	0	4	980	55	5
Side Salad (without dressing)	80	25	3	0	0	5	4	240	11	3
Veggie and Cheese Bare Burrito	580	90	10	4	0	15	20	1950	101	19
Veggie Mix	110	5	0	0	0	0	6	330	24	3

Product	Total Calories	Total Calories from Fat	Total Fat (gm)	Saturated Fat (gm)	Trans Fat (gm)	Cholesterol (mg)	Dietary Fiber (gm)	Sodium (mg)	Carbohydrate (gm)	Protein (gm)

Baskin Robbins®   www.baskinrobbins.com

Product	Total Calories	Total Calories from Fat	Total Fat (gm)	Saturated Fat (gm)	Trans Fat (gm)	Cholesterol (mg)	Dietary Fiber (gm)	Sodium (mg)	Carbohydrate (gm)	Protein (gm)
Rainbow or Orange Sherbet	160	20	2	1.5	0	10	0	40	34	1
Ices (frozen flavors)	130	0	0	0	0	0	0	15	33	0
Low-Fat Cappuccino Blast	220	20	2	1.5	0	10	0	115	45	6
Caramel Turtle Ice Cream	160	35	4	3	0	10	2	137	41	5
Non-fat Frozen Yogurt	150	0	0	0	0	5	0	105	32	6
Pineapple Coconut No Sugar Added Low-Fat Ice Cream	120	20	2	1.5	0	10	0	140	27	5
Raspberry Cheese Louise® Frozen Yogurt	190	30	3.5	2.5	0	10	1	150	35	5

Bob Evans   www.bobevans.com

Product	Total Calories	Total Calories from Fat	Total Fat (gm)	Saturated Fat (gm)	Trans Fat (gm)	Cholesterol (mg)	Dietary Fiber (gm)	Sodium (mg)	Carbohydrate (gm)	Protein (gm)
Bean Soup	205	35	5	2	0	12	7	1111	27	14
Blueberry Hotcake (without syrup)	328	80	9	2	3	0	2	749	55	6
Broccoli Florets	32	10	2	0	0	0	4	29	6	3
Chicken Breast (1 piece, grilled)	232	110	13	3	<1	1	0	635	0	29
Dinner Roll	201	45	5	1	0	9	1	268	34	4
English Muffin	129	10	1	0	0	0	1	298	25	4

Product	Total Calories	Total Calories from Fat	Total Fat (gm)	Saturated Fat (gm)	Trans Fat (gm)	Cholesterol (mg)	Dietary Fiber (gm)	Sodium (mg)	Carbohydrate (gm)	Protein (gm)

Bob Evans (cont.)

Product	Total Calories	Total Calories from Fat	Total Fat (gm)	Saturated Fat (gm)	Trans Fat (gm)	Cholesterol (mg)	Dietary Fiber (gm)	Sodium (mg)	Carbohydrate (gm)	Protein (gm)
Fruit and Yogurt Plate	403	20	2	1	0	5	9	109	93	9
Fruit Cup	150	9	1	0	0	0	4	11	38	2
Fruit Dippers	275	20	2	1	0	5	3	95	61	7
Garden Side Salad (with croutons)	137	35	4	0	0	0	3	347	22	4
Glazed Baby Carrots	83	25	3	1	0	4	4	95	14	1
Grilled Chicken Sandwich	399	135	15	3	1	85	1	945	30	35
Mashed Potatoes	170	55	7	5	0	22	1	458	17	3
Multigrain Hotcake (without syrup)	322	90	10	3	1	0	3	773	52	7
Oatmeal (plain)	172	25	3	0	0	0	4	394	32	6
Raspberry Topping	108	0	0	0	0	0	4	8	27	1
Slow-Roasted Turkey Breast	114	35	4	0	1	47	0	674	1	16
Sugar-free Syrup	39	0	0	0	0	0	0	79	10	0
Texas Toast	120	10	1	0	0	0	1	125	12	2
Vegetable Beef Soup (1 cup)	135	45	5	1	0	14	2	370	14	6

Boston Market®

www.bostonmarket.com

Product	Total Calories	Total Calories from Fat	Total Fat (gm)	Saturated Fat (gm)	Trans Fat (gm)	Cholesterol (mg)	Dietary Fiber (gm)	Sodium (mg)	Carbohydrate (gm)	Protein (gm)
1/4 Rotisserie Chicken (white meat without skin)	210	15	2	.5	0	135	0	640	6	42
Butternut Squash	140	40	4.5	3	0	10	2	35	25	2
Fresh Steamed Vegetables	60	20	2	0	0	0	3	40	8	2
Garlic Dill New Potatoes	140	30	3	1	0	0	3	120	24	3
Hearty Chicken Noodle Soup	170	50	5	1.5	0	60	1	210	17	13
Mashed Potatoes (without gravy)	210	80	9	6	0	25	3	660	29	4
Roasted Sirloin (3 oz.)	290	130	15	6	1	125	0	440	0	39
Rotisserie Chicken Salad (without dressing)	160	10	1	0	0	105	0	520	3	35
Rotisserie Turkey Breast Salad (without dressing)	140	50	6	1	0	25	1	370	1	19
Fresh Vegetable Stuffing	190	70	8	1	0	0	2	580	25	3
Seasonal Fruit Salad	60	5	0	0	0	0	1	20	15	1
Sweet Corn	170	35	4	1	0	0	2	95	37	6
Half Boston Carver Turkey	310	160	18	4.5	0	135	0	940	0	40

Product	Total Calories	Total Calories from Fat	Total Fat (gm)	Saturated Fat (gm)	Trans Fat (gm)	Cholesterol (mg)	Dietary Fiber (gm)	Sodium (mg)	Carbohydrate (gm)	Protein (gm)

Burger King®   www.burgerking.com

Product	Total Calories	Total Calories from Fat	Total Fat (gm)	Saturated Fat (gm)	Trans Fat (gm)	Cholesterol (mg)	Dietary Fiber (gm)	Sodium (mg)	Carbohydrate (gm)	Protein (gm)
BK VEGGIE® Burger	420	160	16	2.5	0	10	7	1100	46	23
TENDERCRISP® Garden Salad (no chicken)	90	50	5	2.5	0	15	3	125	7	5
Hamburger	290	110	12	4.5	0	40	1	560	30	15
MOTTS® Strawberry Flavored Applesauce	90	0	0	0	0	0	<1	0	23	0
Side Garden Salad (without dressing)	15	0	0	0	0	0	1	0	3	1
TENDERGRILL® Chicken Sandwich (without sauce)	400	70	7	1.5	0	70	4	1090	49	37
TENDERGRILL™ Garden Salad (without dressing)	240	90	9	3.5	0	80	4	720	8	33
Whopper Jr.®	370	190	21	6	.5	50	2	570	31	15

Product	Total Calories	Total Calories from Fat	Total Fat (gm)	Saturated Fat (gm)	Trans Fat (gm)	Cholesterol (mg)	Dietary Fiber (gm)	Sodium (mg)	Carbohydrate (gm)	Protein (gm)

Carl's Jr.®   www.carlsjr.com

Product	Total Calories	Total Calories from Fat	Total Fat (gm)	Saturated Fat (gm)	Trans Fat (gm)	Cholesterol (mg)	Dietary Fiber (gm)	Sodium (mg)	Carbohydrate (gm)	Protein (gm)
Charbroiled BBQ Chicken Sandwich	360	40	4.5	1	0	60	4	1150	48	34
Charbroiled Chicken Salad (without dressing)	260	60	7	3.5	0	75	5	710	16	34
Hamburger	460	160	17	6	0	60	2	1060	53	24
Charbroiled Chicken Club	550	210	25	7	0	95	2	1410	43	40
Low-Fat Balsamic Dressing	35	15	1.5	0	0	0	0	480	5	0
Side Salad	50	20	2.5	1.5	0	5	2	60	5	3

Product	Total Calories	Total Calories from Fat	Total Fat (gm)	Saturated Fat (gm)	Trans Fat (gm)	Cholesterol (mg)	Dietary Fiber (gm)	Sodium (mg)	Carbohydrate (gm)	Protein (gm)

Chick-fil-A® www.chickfila.com

Product	Total Calories	Total Calories from Fat	Total Fat (gm)	Saturated Fat (gm)	Trans Fat (gm)	Cholesterol (mg)	Dietary Fiber (gm)	Sodium (mg)	Carbohydrate (gm)	Protein (gm)
Carrot and Raisin Salad	170	50	6	1	0	10	2	110	28	1
Chargrilled Chicken Club (without sauce)	380	100	11	5	0	90	3	1240	33	35
Chargrilled Chicken Cool Wrap®	410	110	12	3.5	0	70	8	1310	46	34
Chargrilled Chicken Garden Salad (without dressing)	180	60	6	3	0	65	3	620	9	22
Chargrilled Chicken Sandwich	270	30	3.5	1	0	65	3	940	33	28
Chick-n-Strips® (4-piece)	310	140	15	3	0	70	1	890	15	28
Chicken Deluxe Sandwich	420	150	16	3.5	0	60	2	1300	39	28
Fat-Free Honey Mustard Dresssing	60	0	0	0	0	0	0	200	14	0
Fruit Cup	70	0	0	0	0	0	2	0	17	1
Light Italian	15	5	.5	0	0	0	0	570	2	0
Reduced-Fat Raspberry Vinaigrette	80	20	2	0	0	0	0	190	15	0
Side Salad (without dressing)	60	25	3	1.5	0	10	2	75	4	3
Southwest Chargrilled Salad (without dressing)	180	60	6	3	0	65	3	620	9	22
Spicy Chicken Cool Wrap®	410	110	12	3.5	0	60	8	1340	44	35

Chili's ®

www.chilis.com

Product	Total Calories	Total Calories from Fat	Total Fat (gm)	Saturated Fat (gm)	Trans Fat (gm)	Cholesterol (mg)	Dietary Fiber (gm)	Sodium (mg)	Carbohydrate (gm)	Protein (gm)
Black Beans with Pico de Gallo	115	0	0	0	0	0	5	640	19	6
Chicken Fajita Pita	450	153	17	3	0	0	3	1750	35	43
Classic Chicken Fajitas (without toppings)	330	99	11	2	0	0	3	2080	23	40
Dinner House Salad (without dressing)	140	63	7	3	0	0	2	190	12	6
Grilled Caribbean Salad (without dressing)	440	90	10	2	0	0	6	1410	51	33
Guacamole (add on)	60	45	15	0	0	0	3	100	3	0
Guiltless Black Bean Burger	650	108	12	2	0	0	26	1940	96	38
Guiltless Chicken Platter	580	72	9	3	0	0	5	2780	85	39
Guiltless Chicken Sandwich	490	72	8	2	0	0	11	2720	63	39
Guiltless Grill® Salmon	480	125	14	3	0	0	3	1080	31	54
Kid's Grilled Chicken Platter	140	25	3	1	0	0	1	620	10	19
Kid's Little Mouth Burger®	280	135	15	5	0	0	1	300	14	20
Rice	160	9	1	0	0	0	1	750	23	3
Sauteed Mushrooms, onions, bell peppers	120	90	10	2	0	0	2	360	6	3

Product	Total Calories	Total Calories from Fat	Total Fat (gm)	Saturated Fat (gm)	Trans Fat (gm)	Cholesterol (mg)	Dietary Fiber (gm)	Sodium (mg)	Carbohydrate (gm)	Protein (gm)

Chili's® (cont.)

Product	Total Calories	Total Calories from Fat	Total Fat (gm)	Saturated Fat (gm)	Trans Fat (gm)	Cholesterol (mg)	Dietary Fiber (gm)	Sodium (mg)	Carbohydrate (gm)	Protein (gm)
Seasonal Grilled Vegetables	50	9	1	1	0	0	3	110	8	4
Firecracker Tilapia	540	126	14	3	0	0	6	1950	63	37
Margarita Grilled Chicken	690	167	18	3	0	9	81	2860	81	48
Steamed Broccoli	80	55	6	1	0	0	3	280	6	3
Sweet Corn-on-the Cob, unbuttered	180	18	2	0	0	0	3	100	55	6

Church's   www.churchs.com

Product	Total Calories	Total Calories from Fat	Total Fat (gm)	Saturated Fat (gm)	Trans Fat (gm)	Cholesterol (mg)	Dietary Fiber (gm)	Sodium (mg)	Carbohydrate (gm)	Protein (gm)
Collard Greens	25	0	0	0	0	0	2	170	5	2
Corn on the Cob	140	27	3	0	0	0	9	15	24	4
Mashed Potatoes and gravy	104	18	2	2	0	<1	1	480	12	2
Original Chicken Breast	200	99	11	3	2	80	1	450	3	22
Original Chicken Leg	110	63	6	2	1	55	0	280	3	10
Spicy Chicken Breast	320	180	20	5	4	75	2	760	12	21
Spicy Fish Fillet	160	81	9	2	2.5	25	1	350	13	7
Spicy Fish Sandwich	320	180	20	4	3	25	2	560	25	10
Spicy Chicken Leg	180	99	11	3	2	65	1	470	8	12

Product	Total Calories	Total Calories from Fat	Total Fat (gm)	Saturated Fat (gm)	Trans Fat (gm)	Cholesterol (mg)	Dietary Fiber (gm)	Sodium (mg)	Carbohydrate (gm)	Protein (gm)

Dairy Queen® www.dairyqueen.com

Product	Total Calories	Total Calories from Fat	Total Fat (gm)	Saturated Fat (gm)	Trans Fat (gm)	Cholesterol (mg)	Dietary Fiber (gm)	Sodium (mg)	Carbohydrate (gm)	Protein (gm)
DQ Chocolate Soft Serve (1/2 cup)	150	45	5	3.5	0	15	0	70	22	4
DQ Fudge Bar (no sugar added)	50	0	0	0	0	0	0	70	13	4
DQ Burger	350	130	14	7	.5	50	1	680	33	17
DQ Vanilla Orange Bar (no sugar added)	66	0	0	0	0	0	0	40	18	2
DQ Vanilla Soft Serve (1/2 cup)	150	45	5	3	0	15	0	70	22	3
Fat-Free Italian Dressing	10	0	0	0	0	0	0	0	0	1
Grilled Chicken Salad (no dressing)	270	100	11	5	0	80	4	1160	92	32
Grilled Chicken Sandwich	400	140	16	2.5	0	55	1	790	32	23
Side Salad (no dressing)	45	0	0	0	0	0	3	50	11	2
Small Chocolate Cone	240	70	7	4.5	0	20	0	115	32	6
Small Chocolate Sundae	280	60	7	4.5	0	20	1	130	49	5
Small Strawberry Sundae	280	60	7	4.5	0	20	1	130	49	5
Small Vanilla Cone	240	70	7	4.5	0	20	0	115	32	6
Starkiss	80	0	0	0	0	0	0	10	21	0

Product	Total Calories	Total Calories from Fat	Total Fat (gm)	Saturated Fat (gm)	Trans Fat (gm)	Cholesterol (mg)	Dietary Fiber (gm)	Sodium (mg)	Carbohydrate (gm)	Protein (gm)
Del Taco								*www.deltaco.com*		
Bean and Cheese Green Burrito	280	70	8	5	0	15	6	1030	38	11
Bean and Cheese Red Burrito	270	70	8	5	0	15	6	1020	38	11
Beans 'n Cheese Cup	220	79	9	3	0	7	11	1139	47	16
Breakfast Burrito	250	100	11	6	0	160	1	520	24	10
Chicken Soft Taco	293	100	11	3	0	35	1	267	18	10
Chicken Taco Del Carbon	170	50	5	1	0	30	2	530	19	12
Half-Pound Green Burrito	430	110	12	9	0	20	13	1690	59	20
Half-Pound Red Burrito	430	110	12	9	0	20	13	1670	65	20
Hamburger	280	80	9	3	0	25	3	640	37	13
Rice Cup	140	20	2	1	0	2	1	910	27	3
Shredded Beef Taco Del Carbon	199	82	11	2	0	28	2	277	17	11
Soft Taco	160	70	8	4	0	20	1	330	16	8
Spicy Chicken Burrito	510	10	17	10	0	5	8	1850	68	28
Taco	160	90	10	4	0	20	1	150	11	7
Veggie Works Burrito	490	160	18	11	0	25	9	1660	69	18

Product	Total Calories	Total Calories from Fat	Total Fat (gm)	Saturated Fat (gm)	Trans Fat (gm)	Cholesterol (mg)	Dietary Fiber (gm)	Sodium (mg)	Carbohydrate (gm)	Protein (gm)

Denny's®   www.dennys.com

Product	Total Calories	Total Calories from Fat	Total Fat (gm)	Saturated Fat (gm)	Trans Fat (gm)	Cholesterol (mg)	Dietary Fiber (gm)	Sodium (mg)	Carbohydrate (gm)	Protein (gm)
Applesauce	60	0	0	0	0	0	1	13	15	0
Blueberry Topping	106	0	0	0	0	0	15	26	0	0
Buttermilk Pancakes (three, without topping)	410	45	5	1	0	0	3	1350	82	9
Cereal (average)	86	0	0	0	0	0	1	278	23	2
Cherry Topping	86	0	0	0	0	0	0	5	21	0
Cinnamon Apple Filling	90	18	2	0	0	0	1	70	19	0
Egg Beaters® Egg Substitute (4 oz.)	56	0	0	0	0	0	0	186	2	11
English Muffin (dry)	150	18	2	0	0	0	2	230	27	5
Grits	80	0	0	0	0	0	0	520	18	2
Ham (grilled slice, honey smoked)	85	27	3	2	0	49	0	1700	6	15
Margarine	87	90	10	2	1.5	0	0	117	0	0
Oatmeal	100	18	2	0	0	0	3	175	18	5
One Egg	120	199	10	3	0	210	0	120	<1	6
Sugar-Free Maple flavored syrup	23	0	0	0	0	0	0	71	9	0

Product	Total Calories	Total Calories from Fat	Total Fat (gm)	Saturated Fat (gm)	Trans Fat (gm)	Cholesterol (mg)	Dietary Fiber (gm)	Sodium (mg)	Carbohydrate (gm)	Protein (gm)

Domino's Pizza ®   *www.dominos.com*

Product	Total Calories	Total Calories from Fat	Total Fat (gm)	Saturated Fat (gm)	Trans Fat (gm)	Cholesterol (mg)	Dietary Fiber (gm)	Sodium (mg)	Carbohydrate (gm)	Protein (gm)
12" Classic Hand-Tossed Cheese	255	90	10	4.5	0	20	0	405	30	11
14" Thin Crust Cheese Pizza (1/8 of pizza)	280	90	9	3.5	0	5	0	0	2	4
14" Thin Crust Veggie Feast (1/8 of pizza)	230	110	12	4.5	0	20	0	0	22	10
Breadstick	130	65	7	1.5	0	0	0	0	14	3

Product	Total Calories	Total Calories from Fat	Total Fat (gm)	Saturated Fat (gm)	Trans Fat (gm)	Cholesterol (mg)	Dietary Fiber (gm)	Sodium (mg)	Carbohydrate (gm)	Protein (gm)
El Pollo Loco								*www.elpolloloco.com*		
BRC Burrito	390	90	10	0	0	15	7	880	25	9
Caesar Pollo Salad (without dressing)	220	63	7	2	0	75	4	580	15	25
Chicken Soft Taco	270	117	13	6	0	75	2	700	19	17
Corn Cobbette	90	9	1	0	0	0	2	0	19	2
Flame-Grilled Chicken Breast	220	81	8	3	0	140	0	620	0	36
Flame-Grilled Chicken Breast (skinless)	180	36	4	1	0	110	0	560	0	35
Flame-Grilled Chicken Leg	90	36	4	1	0	70	0	170	0	12
Flame-Grilled Chicken Thigh	220	135	15	5	0	180	0	320	0	12
Garden Salad (without dressing)	120	63	7	4	0	15	2	290	9	5
Gravy	10	0	0	0	0	0	0	150	0	0
Light Italian Dressing	20	9	1	0	0	0	0	770	2	0
Lite Creamy Cilantro Dressing	70	45	5	1	0	5	0	400	6	1
Mashed Potatoes	100	9	1	0	0	0	2	350	20	2
Pinto Beans	140	0	0	0	0	0	7	330	25	9
Pollo Bowl (without dressing)	540	36	4	1	0	70	11	1590	85	37
Spanish Rice	160	9	1	0	0	0	1	420	34	3
Taco Al Carbon	150	45	5	2	0	40	2	290	17	11
Steamed Vegetables (with no margarine)	35	0	0	0	0	0	1	35	8	2

Product	Total Calories	Total Calories from Fat	Total Fat (gm)	Saturated Fat (gm)	Trans Fat (gm)	Cholesterol (mg)	Dietary Fiber (gm)	Sodium (mg)	Carbohydrate (gm)	Protein (gm)

Fazoli's®

www.fazolis.com

Product	Total Calories	Total Calories from Fat	Total Fat (gm)	Saturated Fat (gm)	Trans Fat (gm)	Cholesterol (mg)	Dietary Fiber (gm)	Sodium (mg)	Carbohydrate (gm)	Protein (gm)
Garlic Breadstick	150	60	7	1.5	0	0	0	290	20	3
Caesar Side Salad	40	20	2	1	0	5	2	70	4	4
Cheese Pizza	270	100	11	4	.5	25	2	700	31	13
Chicken and Fruit Salad	220	15	1.5	0	0	55	4	700	28	23
Dry Breadstick	100	15	2	0	0	0	0	160	20	3
Fat-Free Honey Mustard Dressing	60	0	0	0	0	0	1	350	15	0
Fat-Free Italian Dressing	25	0	0	0	0	0	6	390	6	0
Garden Side Salad (without dressing)	25	5	0	0	0	0	3	30	4	2
Panini Grilled Chicken Sandwich	540	162	18	.5	0	80	3	1360	56	35
Penne with Marinara (small)	450	25	2.5	0	0	0	7	770	88	15
Spaghetti in Meat Sauce (with broccoli)	500	60	7	1.5	0	10	7	1020	87	20
Spaghetti with Marinara (small)	450	25	2.5	0	0	0	7	770	88	15

Product	Total Calories	Total Calories from Fat	Total Fat (gm)	Saturated Fat (gm)	Trans Fat (gm)	Cholesterol (mg)	Dietary Fiber (gm)	Sodium (mg)	Carbohydrate (gm)	Protein (gm)

Golden Corral ®   www.goldencorral.com

Product	Total Calories	Total Calories from Fat	Total Fat (gm)	Saturated Fat (gm)	Trans Fat (gm)	Cholesterol (mg)	Dietary Fiber (gm)	Sodium (mg)	Carbohydrate (gm)	Protein (gm)
Black-eyed Peas	149	10	1	0	0	0	0	500	4	1
Cajun Style Fish Fillet	210	80	9.4	0	0	0	0	650	18.5	12.9
Cajun Whitefish	110	65	7	0	0	0	0	859	0	10
Carved Salmon Fillet	138	80	9	0	0	0	0	274	0	11
Chicken Gumbo	70	15	1.5	0	0	10	1	740	10	5
Chicken Noodle	100	25	2.5	.5	0	55	1	1240	12	6
Clam Chowder	140	55	6	2	0	10	1	1110	17	4
Corn-on-the-Cob	106	20	2	0	0	0	0	20	22	3
Escalloped Apples	180	20	2	.5	0	0	0	20	27	2
Fat-Free Thousand Island Dressing	40	0	0	0	0	0	.5	250	9	0
Fat-Free Ranch Dressing	40	0	0	0	0	0	0	290	2	0
Green Beans	34	0	0	0	0	0	0	415	6	1
Grilled Pork Chop or Loin slices	119	35	4	0	0	0	0	153	0	19
Kaiser Roll	160	15	1.5	.5	0	0	1	350	31	6
Lite Olive Oil Vinaigrette	60	55	6	1	0	0	0	230	0	0
Marinated Vegetables	47	20	2	0	0	0	0	140	5	1
Mashed Potato	120	55	6	1.5	0	0	1	260	16	2
Ranch Style BBQ Beans	130	25	3	1	0	0	6	540	40	1

Golden Corral® (cont.)

Product	Total Calories	Total Calories from Fat	Total Fat (gm)	Saturated Fat (gm)	Trans Fat (gm)	Cholesterol (mg)	Dietary Fiber (gm)	Sodium (mg)	Carbohydrate (gm)	Protein (gm)
Roast Beef	180	90	10	3.5	0	65	0	135	1	23
Skillet Cornbread	120	25	2.5	.5	0	15	1	320	22	2
Smoked Ham	80	20	2	1	0	30	0	560	1	10
Spinach	20	0	0	0	0	0	0	115	11	4
Steamed Broccoli	25	5	<.5	0	0	0	0	170	5	3
Steamed Cabbage	60	45	5	0	0	0	0	80	0	0
Steamed Carrots	79	45	5	0	0	0	0	97	6	0
Steamed Cauliflower	13	0	0	0	0	0	0	162	6	0
Sweet Potato	137	0	0	0	0	0	0	17	32	2
Timberline Chili	270	110	12	4.5	0	40	5	930	23	19
Turkey Breast	70	25	3	1	0	30	0	340	1	10
Vegetable Beef Soup	100	15	1.5	.5	0	.5	2	1230	17	5
Vegetable Trio	25	0	0	0	0	0	0	170	5	1
Yams and Apples	160	20	.2	.5	0	0	1	110	35	1

Product	Total Calories	Total Calories from Fat	Total Fat (gm)	Saturated Fat (gm)	Trans Fat (gm)	Cholesterol (mg)	Dietary Fiber (gm)	Sodium (mg)	Carbohydrate (gm)	Protein (gm)

Hardee's ®   www.hardees.com

Product	Total Calories	Total Calories from Fat	Total Fat (gm)	Saturated Fat (gm)	Trans Fat (gm)	Cholesterol (mg)	Dietary Fiber (gm)	Sodium (mg)	Carbohydrate (gm)	Protein (gm)
BBQ Sauce	45	0	0	0	0	0	1	290	10	1
Charbroiled BBQ Chicken Sandwich	320	50	6	1	0	50	3	1200	43	33
Hamburger	310	110	12	4	0	35	1	560	36	14
Mashed Potatoes (small)	90	15	2	0	0	0	0	410	17	1
Pancake Platter	300	45	5	1	0	25	2	830	55	8
Sweet and Sour Sauce	45	0	0	0	0	0	0	85	10	0

Jack in the Box® www.jackinthebox.com

Product	Total Calories	Total Calories from Fat	Total Fat (gm)	Saturated Fat (gm)	Trans Fat (gm)	Cholesterol (mg)	Dietary Fiber (gm)	Sodium (mg)	Carbohydrate (gm)	Protein (gm)
Asian Chicken Salad (without dressing)	160	15	1.5	0	0	65	5	380	18	22
Breakfast Jack®	290	110	12	4.5	0	220	1	760	29	17
Chicken Fajita Pita	280	80	9	3.5	0	60	2	1110	30	21
Chicken Sandwich	400	190	21	4.5	2.5	35	2	730	38	15
Fruit Cup	90	5	0	0	0	0	0	20	22	1
Hamburger	280	110	12	4.5	.5	30	1	580	30	14
Lite Ranch Dressing	190	170	18	3	0	25	0	700	3	1
Low-Fat Balsamic Dressing	40	20	2	0	0	0	0	600	6	0
Side Salad (without dressing)	50	25	3	1.5	0	10	2	260	5	3

Kentucky Fried Chicken ™ www.kfc.com

Product	Total Calories	Total Calories from Fat	Total Fat (gm)	Saturated Fat (gm)	Trans Fat (gm)	Cholesterol (mg)	Dietary Fiber (gm)	Sodium (mg)	Carbohydrate (gm)	Protein (gm)
BBQ Baked Beans	220	10	1	0	0	0	7	730	45	8
Corn on the Cob (3")	70	15	1.5	.5	0	0	3	53	13	2
Crispy Strips	350	170	19	3.5	0	70	0	1190	16	29
Green Beans	50	15	1.5	0	0	5	2	570	7	2
Honey BBQ Sandwich	280	30	3.5	1	0	60	3	780	40	22
House Side Salad (without dressing)	15	0	0	0	0	0	1	10	2	1
Lil' Bucket Strawberry Shortcake	210	70	7	5	0	10	1	125	33	2
Mashed Potatoes (with gravy)	140	45	5	1	.5	0	1	560	20	2
Mashed Potatoes (without gravy)	110	35	4	1	0	0	1	320	17	2
Original Recipe Breast (without skin or breading)	140	20	2	0	0	65	0	520	1	29
Original Recipe Drumstick	130	70	8	2	0	65	0	350	2	12
Oven Roasted Twister (without sauce)	330	70	7	2.5	0	50	3	1120	39	28
Roasted BLT Salad (without dressing)	200	60	6	2	0	65	4	880	8	29
Seasoned Rice	150	10	1	0	0	0	2	630	32	4
Sweet Life Oatmeal Raisin cookie	150	50	5	2.5	0	5	1	135	24	2
Teddy Grahams® Graham snacks	90	25	3	.5	0	0	1	95	15	1
Tender Roast® Sandwich (without sauce)	300	40	4.5	1.5	0	70	2	1060	28	37

Product	Total Calories	Total Calories from Fat	Total Fat (gm)	Saturated Fat (gm)	Trans Fat (gm)	Cholesterol (mg)	Dietary Fiber (gm)	Sodium (mg)	Carbohydrate (gm)	Protein (gm)

Little Caesar's® www.littlecaesars.com

Product	Total Calories	Total Calories from Fat	Total Fat (gm)	Saturated Fat (gm)	Trans Fat (gm)	Cholesterol (mg)	Dietary Fiber (gm)	Sodium (mg)	Carbohydrate (gm)	Protein (gm)
14" Round Cheese Pizza (1/10 pizza)	200	60	3.5	3	0	15	1	340	2	10
14" Round Pepperoni Pizza (1/10 pizza)	230	80	9	4.5	0	20	1	420	25	11
14" Thin Crust Cheese Pizza (1/10 pizza)	160	66	7.3	3.5	0	15	0	210	14	8
14" Thin Crust Pepperoni Pizza (1/10 pizza)	180	80	8.8	4.5	0	20	0	320	14	9
Caesar Salad (no dressing)	90	27	2.9	1	0	0	3	190	12	4
Crazy Bread® (1 slice)	100	25	3	.5	0	1	0	150	15	3
Crazy Sauce® (4 oz.)	45	0	0	0	0	0	3	260	10	2
Fat-Free Italian Dressing (1 package)	25	0	0	0	0	0	0	390	5	0
Medium Deep Dish Cheese (1/8 pizza)	320	120	13	5	0	25	1	490	38	14
Medium Deep Dish Pepperoni (1/8 pizza)	360	140	16	6	0	30	1	610	38	16
Tossed Salad	100	28	3.1	1	0	0	3	190	15	2

Product	Total Calories	Total Calories from Fat	Total Fat (gm)	Saturated Fat (gm)	Trans Fat (gm)	Cholesterol (mg)	Dietary Fiber (gm)	Sodium (mg)	Carbohydrate (gm)	Protein (gm)
Lone Star Steakhouse					*www.lonestarsteakhouse.com*					
El Paso Salad with Mesquite-Grilled Shrimp	207	27	3	1	0	297	0	290	2	39
Grilled Chicken (6 oz.)	186	22	2.4	.6	0	96	0	108	0	39
Steamed Vegetables	71	9	1	0	0	0	22	912	14	5
Texas Rice	80	18	2	1	0	6	1	207	12	2

Product	Total Calories	Total Calories from Fat	Total Fat (gm)	Saturated Fat (gm)	Trans Fat (gm)	Cholesterol (mg)	Dietary Fiber (gm)	Sodium (mg)	Carbohydrate (gm)	Protein (gm)

McDonald's ®   www.mcdonalds.com

Product	Total Calories	Total Calories from Fat	Total Fat (gm)	Saturated Fat (gm)	Trans Fat (gm)	Cholesterol (mg)	Dietary Fiber (gm)	Sodium (mg)	Carbohydrate (gm)	Protein (gm)
Apple Dippers with Low-Fat Caramel Dip	105	5	.5	0	0	5	0	35	23	0
Asian Salad (without chicken)	150	70	7	.5	0	0	5	35	15	8
Asian Salad (with grilled chicken)	300	90	10	1	0	65	5	890	23	32
Bacon Ranch Salad (with grilled chicken)	260	90	9	4	0	90	3	1010	12	33
Bacon Ranch Salad (without chicken)	140	70	7	3.5	0	25	3	300	10	9
Caesar Salad (with grilled chicken)	220	60	6	3	0	75	3	890	12	30
Egg McMuffin®	300	10	12	5	0	260	2	820	30	18
English Muffin	140	15	1.5	0	0	0	2	260	27	5
Fruit and Yogurt Parfait	160	20	2	1	0	5	1	85	31	4
Fruit and Walnut Salad	210	70	8	1.5	0	5	2	60	31	4
Grape Jam	35	0	0	0	0	0	0	0	9	0
Hamburger	250	80	9	3.5	.5	25	2	520	31	12
Honey Mustard Snack Wrap™ (with grilled chicken)	260	80	9	3.5	0	46	1	800	27	18
Newman's Own® Low-Fat Balsamic Vinaigrette	40	25	3	0	0	0	0	730	4	0

Product	Total Calories	Total Calories from Fat	Total Fat (gm)	Saturated Fat (gm)	Trans Fat (gm)	Cholesterol (mg)	Dietary Fiber (gm)	Sodium (mg)	Carbohydrate (gm)	Protein (gm)

McDonald's® (cont.)

Product	Total Calories	Total Calories from Fat	Total Fat (gm)	Saturated Fat (gm)	Trans Fat (gm)	Cholesterol (mg)	Dietary Fiber (gm)	Sodium (mg)	Carbohydrate (gm)	Protein (gm)
Newman's Own® Low-Fat Family Recipe	60	20	2.5	0	0	0	0	730	8	1
Premium Grilled Chicken Classic Sandwich	420	90	10	2	0	70	3	1190	51	32
Ranch Snack Wrap™ (with Grilled Chicken)	270	90	10	4	0	45	1	830	26	18
Scrambled Eggs	170	100	11	4	0	520	0	180	1	15
Southwest Salad (without chicken)	140	40	4.5	2	0	10	6	150	20	6
Southwest Salad (with grilled chicken)	320	90	9	3	0	70	7	970	30	30
Strawberry Preserves	35	0	0	0	0	0	0	0	9	0

Old Country Buffet ®   www.oldcountrybuffet.com

Product	Total Calories	Total Calories from Fat	Total Fat (gm)	Saturated Fat (gm)	Trans Fat (gm)	Cholesterol (mg)	Dietary Fiber (gm)	Sodium (mg)	Carbohydrate (gm)	Protein (gm)
California Coleslaw (1 spoon)	100	0	0	0	0	0	1	8	24	1
Carved Ham (3 oz.)	140	81	9	3	0	45	0	970	1	13
Carved Peppered Pork Loin (3 oz.)	160	72	8	5	0	60	0	810	0	23
Carved Roast Turkey (3 oz.)	170	72	8	2.5	0	70	0	60	0	24
Chicken and Dumplings (1 spoon)	170	54	6	1	0	30	<1	530	7	11
Chicken Noodle Soup (4 oz. ladle)	80	20	2	.5	0	20	<1	300	8	6
Chicken Rice Soup (4 oz. ladle)	60	15	1.5	.5	0	0	1	300	8	6
Chili Bean Soup (4 oz. ladle)	80	35	3.5	1.5	0	15	1	340	9	7
Cucumber Tomato Salad (1 spoon)	30	10	1	0	0	0	1	390	4	<1
Dinner Roll	130	45	5	1	0	0	1	280	23	2
English Muffin	60	5	.5	0	0	0	<1	200	13	2
Fish Patties (2-1/2 oz. piece)	180	100	9	1.5	0	20	0	510	17	8
Fried Fish (1 piece)	90	39	4.5	1	0	10	0	210	10	3
Green Beans (1 spoon)	15	0	0	0	0	0	1	340	3	<1
Grits (4 oz. ladle)	60	0	0	0	0	0	0	125	13	1
Low-Fat Italian Dressing (1 ladle)	25	20	0	0	0	0	0	430	2	0

Product	Total Calories	Total Calories from Fat	Total Fat (gm)	Saturated Fat (gm)	Trans Fat (gm)	Cholesterol (mg)	Dietary Fiber (gm)	Sodium (mg)	Carbohydrate (gm)	Protein (gm)

Old Country Buffet® (cont.)

Product	Total Calories	Total Calories from Fat	Total Fat (gm)	Saturated Fat (gm)	Trans Fat (gm)	Cholesterol (mg)	Dietary Fiber (gm)	Sodium (mg)	Carbohydrate (gm)	Protein (gm)
Navy Bean with Ham (4 oz. ladle)	50	5	<1	0	0	0	4	410	10	5
Oatmeal (4 oz. ladle)	60	12	9.5	0	0	0	2	110	12	2
Pancake (1; without butter or syrup)	130	45	5	1	0	0	<1	280	19	2
Pickled Beets (1 spoon)	100	0	0	0	0	0	2	125	25	<1
Poached Egg	70	45	5	1.5	0	210	0	150	0	6
Reduced-Fat Ranch Dressing (1 ladle)	60	60	6	1	0	1-	0	230	2	<1
Scrambled Eggs (1 spoon)	120	90	10	2.5	0	100	0	80	<1	7
Soft Serve Frozen Yogurt, nonfat, strawberry	90	0	0	0	0	0	0	55	23	3
Soft Serve Frozen Yogurt, nonfat, vanilla	100	0	0	0	0	0	0	70	21	3
Spaghetti (1 spoon)	130	22	2.5	.5	0	0	1	90	23	3
Spring Mix Salads	5	0	0	0	0	0	1	5	0	<1
Steamed Carrots (1 spoon)	40	2.5	.5	0	0	0	3	65	7	<1
Steamed Corn (1 spoon)	90	20	2.5	.5	0	0	2	210	17	3
Strawberry Peach Banana salad (1 spoon)	70	0	0	0	0	0	1	17	14	<1

Product	Total Calories	Total Calories from Fat	Total Fat (gm)	Saturated Fat (gm)	Trans Fat (gm)	Cholesterol (mg)	Dietary Fiber (gm)	Sodium (mg)	Carbohydrate (gm)	Protein (gm)

Old Country Buffet® (cont.)

Product	Total Calories	Total Calories from Fat	Total Fat (gm)	Saturated Fat (gm)	Trans Fat (gm)	Cholesterol (mg)	Dietary Fiber (gm)	Sodium (mg)	Carbohydrate (gm)	Protein (gm)
Tossed Green Salad (1 cup)	5	0	0	0	0	0	1	5	1	<1
Traditional Baked Chicken breast	270	110	12	3.5	0	125	0	270	0	40
Traditional Baked Chicken drumstick	130	81	9	25	0	45	0	160	0	13
Vegetable Medley (1 cup)	50	35	4.5	1.5	0	0	1	160	2	1
Waffle (1; without butter or syrup)	120	30	3	.5	0	0	<1	420	19	3
Wild Rice Vegetable Pilaf (1 spoon)	100	15	1.5	0	0	0	<1	370	17	3

Product	Total Calories	Total Calories from Fat	Total Fat (gm)	Saturated Fat (gm)	Trans Fat (gm)	Cholesterol (mg)	Dietary Fiber (gm)	Sodium (mg)	Carbohydrate (gm)	Protein (gm)

On the Border®　　　　　　　　　　　　www.ontheborder.com

Product	Total Calories	Total Calories from Fat	Total Fat (gm)	Saturated Fat (gm)	Trans Fat (gm)	Cholesterol (mg)	Dietary Fiber (gm)	Sodium (mg)	Carbohydrate (gm)	Protein (gm)
Black Bean and Corn Relish (2 oz.)	70	40	4	0	0	0	1	160	6	1
Black Beans	180	65	7	2	0	0	6	690	19	8
Chicken Salsa Fresca	510	100	11	4	0	0	6	600	48	49
Chili Con Carne Sauce	70	30	3	0	0	0	1	360	6	4
Corn Tortilla (2)	140	20	2	0	0	0	3	126	30	4
Fat-Free Balsamic Vinaigrette	50	0	0	0	0	0	0	610	10	0
Grilled Chicken Fajita Tacos	630	130	14	2	0	0	21	1540	97	37
Guacamole (1 scoop)	60	45	5	1	0	0	2	200	4	1
House Salad	170	90	10	4	0	0	4	110	15	6
Jalapeno-BBQ Salmon	530	170	18	2.5	0	0	9	1600	44	47
Original Mesquite-Grilled Chicken Fajitas	440	170	18	3	0	0	4	1870	20	48
Pico de Gallo	20	9	1	0	0	0	1	120	2	0
Pico Shrimp Tacos	640	10	0	3	0	0	20	1140	94	38
Salsa	25	9	1	0	0	0	2	160	3	0
Salsa Fresca	20	0	0	0	0	0	.5	0	3	1
Soft Taco Chicken (1)	250	100	11	5	0	0	1	910	20	13
Vegetables (grilled)	50	10	1	0	0	0	3	190	8	2

Product	Total Calories	Total Calories from Fat	Total Fat (gm)	Saturated Fat (gm)	Trans Fat (gm)	Cholesterol (mg)	Dietary Fiber (gm)	Sodium (mg)	Carbohydrate (gm)	Protein (gm)

Panda Express

www.pandaexpress.com

Product	Total Calories	Total Calories from Fat	Total Fat (gm)	Saturated Fat (gm)	Trans Fat (gm)	Cholesterol (mg)	Dietary Fiber (gm)	Sodium (mg)	Carbohydrate (gm)	Protein (gm)
Broccoli Beef (5.5 oz.)	150	80	7	1.5	0	25	4	510	11	11
Chow Mein (8 oz.)	390	110	12	2	0	0	7	1020	59	11
Egg Flower Soup (12 oz.)	88	22	2.2	0	0	55	0	895	16	2
Hot and Sour Soup (12 oz.)	110	35	3.5	1	0	85	2	1370	14	5
Mandarin Chicken (5.5 oz.)	250	90	10	3	0	145	0	1150	8	31
Mixed Veggies	70	35	4	.5	0	0	<1	170	6	4
Steamed Rice	380	20	2.5	.5	0	0	4	30	81	9
Sweet and Sour Sauce (1.5 oz.)	80	0	0	0	0	0	0	135	19	0
Tangy Shrimp (5.5 oz.)	150	50	5	1	0	85	2	550	16	9
Veggie Spring Roll (1 roll)	90	60	7	1	0	0	3	100	8	2

Product	Total Calories	Total Calories from Fat	Total Fat (gm)	Saturated Fat (gm)	Trans Fat (gm)	Cholesterol (mg)	Dietary Fiber (gm)	Sodium (mg)	Carbohydrate (gm)	Protein (gm)

Panera Bread®   www.panerabread.com

Product	Total Calories	Total Calories from Fat	Total Fat (gm)	Saturated Fat (gm)	Trans Fat (gm)	Cholesterol (mg)	Dietary Fiber (gm)	Sodium (mg)	Carbohydrate (gm)	Protein (gm)
Artisan Country Bread (2 oz.)	120	0	0	0	0	0	1	300	25	5
Artisan Three Cheese Bread (2 oz.)	130	20	2	1	0	5	1	290	23	5
Chicken Noodle Soup	100	20	2	0	0	15	1	1080	15	5
Chicken Tomesto Sandwich on Three Cheese Bread (half)	310	80	8	2	0	40	3	760	40	21
Fresh Fruit Cup	70	0	0	0	0	0	1	15	19	1
Grilled Salmon Salad (half portion)	170	60	7	1	0	25	3	410	16	11
Kid's Deli Sandwich (smoked turkey)	350	100	12	7	0	60	3	1440	36	25
Low-Fat Southwest Tomato and Roasted Corn Soup	110	25	3	0	0	0	4	700	20	3
Low-Fat Vegetarian Black Bean Soup	160	10	1	0	0	0	11	820	31	9
Low-Fat Vegetarian Garden Soup	90	5	.5	0	0	0	2	860	17	4
Mediterranean Veggie Sandwich (half portion)	300	60	6	1.5	0	5	5	730	50	11
Rosemary and Onion Focaccia (2 oz.)	150	45	5	1.5	0	5	1	300	22	5
Smoked Turkey Breast Sandwich on Sourdough (half)	230	80	8	1.5	0	30	2	840	24	15
Whole Grain Bread (2 oz.)	140	10	1	0	0	0	3	320	27	6

Papa John's®

www.papajohns.com

Product	Total Calories	Total Calories from Fat	Total Fat (gm)	Saturated Fat (gm)	Trans Fat (gm)	Cholesterol (mg)	Dietary Fiber (gm)	Sodium (mg)	Carbohydrate (gm)	Protein (gm)
14" Hawaiian Barbeque Chicken (1/8 pizza)	340	100	11	3.5	0	30	2	960	46	16
14" Original Crust Cheese Pizza (1/8 pizza)	300	100	11	3.5	0	20	2	750	39	13
14" Original Crust Garden Fresh Pizza (1/8 pizza)	280	80	9	2.5	0	30	2	940	38	15
14" Original Crust Pepperoni Pizza (1/8 pizza)	210	120	13	4	0	20	2	800	38	13
14" Thin Crust Cheese Pizza (1/8 pizza)	240	120	13	3.5	0	20	1	550	22	10
14" Thin Crust Garden Fresh Pizza (1/8 pizza)	210	100	11	2.5	0	15	2	430	23	8
14" Thin Crust Pepperoni Pizza (1/8 pizza)	260	140	15	4.5	0	20	1	580	23	10
BBQ Dipping Sauce (1 oz.)	40	0	0	0	0	0	0	240	11	0
Breadstick (1)	140	20	2	0	0	0	1	260	26	4
Pizza Dipping Sauce (1 oz.)	20	0	0	0	0	0	0	140	3	0

Product	Total Calories	Total Calories from Fat	Total Fat (gm)	Saturated Fat (gm)	Trans Fat (gm)	Cholesterol (mg)	Dietary Fiber (gm)	Sodium (mg)	Carbohydrate (gm)	Protein (gm)

Pizza Hut ®   www.pizzahut.com

Product	Total Calories	Total Calories from Fat	Total Fat (gm)	Saturated Fat (gm)	Trans Fat (gm)	Cholesterol (mg)	Dietary Fiber (gm)	Sodium (mg)	Carbohydrate (gm)	Protein (gm)
14" Cheese Hand Tossed Crust (1/8 pizza)	340	130	14	7	1.5	35	2	900	36	17
14" Cheese Pan Pizza (1/8 pizza)	390	170	19	7	0	35	2	800	38	16
14" Cheese Thin Crust (1/8 pizza)	280	110	12	6	0	35	1	810	30	14
14" Fit n' Delicious™ Pizza—Diced Chicken, Mushrooms and Jalapeno	230	60	6	2.5	0	25	2	1010	30	13
14" Fit n' Delicious™ Pizza—Ham, Red Onion and Mushroom	230	60	7	2.5	0	20	2	820	31	11
14" Fit n' Delicious™ Pizza—Ham, Pineapple and Diced Red Tomato	230	60	6	2.5	0	20	1	830	32	11
14" Fit n' Delicious™ Pizza—Diced Red Tomato, Mushroom and Jalapeno	210	50	6	2.5	0	10	2	870	36	10
14" Fit n' Delicious™ Pizza—Green Pepper, Red Onion and Diced Red Tomato	210	50	6	2.5	0	10	2	580	32	8
14" Fit n' Delicious™ Pizza—Diced Chicken, Red Onion and Green Pepper	230	60	6	2.5	0	25	2	730	32	13

Product	Total Calories	Total Calories from Fat	Total Fat (gm)	Saturated Fat (gm)	Trans Fat (gm)	Cholesterol (mg)	Dietary Fiber (gm)	Sodium (mg)	Carbohydrate (gm)	Protein (gm)

Pizza Hut ® (cont.)

Product	Total Calories	Total Calories from Fat	Total Fat (gm)	Saturated Fat (gm)	Trans Fat (gm)	Cholesterol (mg)	Dietary Fiber (gm)	Sodium (mg)	Carbohydrate (gm)	Protein (gm)
14" Pepperoni Hand Tossed Crust (1/8 pizza)	360	150	16	7	1.5	40	2	1010	35	17
14" Pepperoni Pan Pizza (1/8 pizza)	400	190	21	7	0	40	2	900	37	16
14" Pepperoni Thin Crust (1/8 pizza)	300	130	14	6	0	40	1	920	29	14
14" Veggie Lover's® Hand Tossed Crust (1/8 pizza)	310	100	12	5	1.5	25	2	840	37	14
14" Veggie Lover's® Pan Pizza (1/8 pizza)	350	150	16	6	0	25	2	730	39	14
14" Veggie Lover's® Thin Crust (1/8 pizza)	260	90	10	4.5	0	25	2	770	31	12

Product	Total Calories	Total Calories from Fat	Total Fat (gm)	Saturated Fat (gm)	Trans Fat (gm)	Cholesterol (mg)	Dietary Fiber (gm)	Sodium (mg)	Carbohydrate (gm)	Protein (gm)

Popeye's ®   www.popeyes.com

Product	Total Calories	Total Calories from Fat	Total Fat (gm)	Saturated Fat (gm)	Trans Fat (gm)	Cholesterol (mg)	Dietary Fiber (gm)	Sodium (mg)	Carbohydrate (gm)	Protein (gm)
Cajun Rice	170	55	6	2	0	60	2	530	22	8
Corn on the Cob	190	20	2	.5	0	0	4	0	37	6
Crawfish Etoufee	180	45	5	1	0	48	2	640	25	7
Deluxe Chicken Sandwich (without mayonnaise)	480	135	15	6	.5	55	3	1290	54	33
Green Beans	70	10	1	0	0	5	2	400	14	2
Mashed Potatoes (without gravy)	100	30	3	1	.5	0	<1	380	17	1
Mild Chicken Breast (skinless and breading)	120	20	2	1	0	120	0	540	0	24
Mild Chicken Leg (skinless and breading removed)	50	20	2	.5	0	85	0	190	0	9
Spicy Chicken Breast (skinless and breading removed)	120	20	2	1	0	112	<1	380	<1	25
Spicy Chicken Leg (skinless and breading removed)	50	15	1.5	.5	0	60	0	135	0	9

Product	Total Calories	Total Calories from Fat	Total Fat (gm)	Saturated Fat (gm)	Trans Fat (gm)	Cholesterol (mg)	Dietary Fiber (gm)	Sodium (mg)	Carbohydrate (gm)	Protein (gm)

Rubio's Fresh Mexican Grill ®   www.rubios.com

Product	Total Calories	Total Calories from Fat	Total Fat (gm)	Saturated Fat (gm)	Trans Fat (gm)	Cholesterol (mg)	Dietary Fiber (gm)	Sodium (mg)	Carbohydrate (gm)	Protein (gm)
Black Beans	130	10	1.5	.5	0	5	5	330	25	14
Carne Asada Street Taco	130	50	6	2	0	20	1	360	10	8
Carnitas (with corn tortillas)	210	80	9	3.5	0	0	2	90	30	12
Chicken Street Taco	110	30	3.5	.5	0	30	1	240	10	11
Fat-Free Serrano Grape Dressing	40	0	0	0	0	0	0	135	9	0
HealthMex® Chicken Salad	270	25	3	0	0	70	7	1020	70	36
HealthMex® Chicken Taco	150	15	3	0	0	30	2	350	21	12
HealthMex® Mahi Mahi Taco	150	15	2	0	0	15	2	180	21	12
Pinto Beans	130	10	1.5	.5	0	5	1	330	25	4
Rice (small)	100	45	5	0	0	0	1	140	2	1
Wet Burrito	120	70	8	4.5	0	15	6	520	0	4

Schlotzsky's ®   *www.schlotzskys.com*

Product	Total Calories	Total Calories from Fat	Total Fat (gm)	Saturated Fat (gm)	Trans Fat (gm)	Cholesterol (mg)	Dietary Fiber (gm)	Sodium (mg)	Carbohydrate (gm)	Protein (gm)
Asian Chicken Wrap	505	101	11	0	0	43	5	2018	79	44
Caesar Salad	103	42	5	0	0	6	3	289	10	6
Fruit Salad	100	5	0	0	0	0	2	35	25	1
Garden Salad	51	13	1	0	0	0	4	291	12	3
Greek Salad	137	75	8	0	0	29	4	655	13	7
Grilled Chicken Caesar Salad	221	68	8	0	0	65	3	759	12	53
Hearty Vegetable Beef Soup (1 cup)	109	45	5	0	0	15	2	1020	12	6
Homestyle Tuna Wrap	480	177	20	0	0	50	4	1199	55	21
Mediterranean Tuna Wrap	440	126	14	0	0	33	5	1304	57	21
Medium Chipotle Grilled Chicken	578	116	13	0	0	92	4	1316	76	80
Medium Dijon Chicken	614	106	12	0	0	86	8	2126	86	86
Medium Fresh Veggie	483	107	12	0	0	23	6	1153	77	18
Medium Grilled Chicken breast	545	62	7	0	0	86	5	1702	80	80
Medium Smoked Turkey breast	500	66	7	0	0	59	4	1806	76	33
Medium Turkey and guacamole	552	107	12	0	0	52	6	1955	80	34
Old Fashioned Chicken Noodle Soup (1 cup)	90	14	2	0	0	55	1	1243	11	7

Product	Total Calories	Total Calories from Fat	Total Fat (gm)	Saturated Fat (gm)	Trans Fat (gm)	Cholesterol (mg)	Dietary Fiber (gm)	Sodium (mg)	Carbohydrate (gm)	Protein (gm)

Schlotzsky's® (cont.)

Product	Total Calories	Total Calories from Fat	Total Fat (gm)	Saturated Fat (gm)	Trans Fat (gm)	Cholesterol (mg)	Dietary Fiber (gm)	Sodium (mg)	Carbohydrate (gm)	Protein (gm)
Side Salad	26	6	1	0	0	0	2	236	7	1
Small Chipotle Grilled Chicken	405	92	10	0	0	69	3	956	50	56
Small Dijon Chicken	391	65	7	0	0	46	5	1539	54	30
Small Fresh Veggie	355	91	10	0	0	23	4	772	52	14
Small Grilled Chicken breast	372	42	5	0	0	59	3	1121	55	55
Small Smoked Turkey breast	345	46	5	0	0	40	2	1240	53	23
Small Turkey and guacamole	364	60	7	0	0	36	4	1300	54	22
Timberline Chili (1 cup)	227	71	8	0	1	35	8	890	26	15
Vegetable Soup (1 cup)	85	9	1	0	0	0	4	900	19	2

Product	Total Calories	Total Calories from Fat	Total Fat (gm)	Saturated Fat (gm)	Trans Fat (gm)	Cholesterol (mg)	Dietary Fiber (gm)	Sodium (mg)	Carbohydrate (gm)	Protein (gm)

Sonic®   www.sonicdrivein.com

Product	Total Calories	Total Calories from Fat	Total Fat (gm)	Saturated Fat (gm)	Trans Fat (gm)	Cholesterol (mg)	Dietary Fiber (gm)	Sodium (mg)	Carbohydrate (gm)	Protein (gm)
Fat-Free Golden Italian Dressing	50	0	0	0	0	0	0	600	13	0
Grilled Chicken on Ciabatta	340	100	12	2.5	.5	75	2	990	32	27
Grilled Chicken Salad	310	120	13	6	1	95	4	1070	19	29
Grilled Chicken Wrap	380	100	11	2.5	1	75	4	1300	44	27
Jr. Burger	310	130	15	5	.5	35	2	610	30	15
Original Light Ranch Dressing	120	60	7	1	0	15	0	740	14	1
Sante Fe Chicken Salad	380	140	15	7	1	100	6	1180	29	30

Product	Total Calories	Total Calories from Fat	Total Fat (gm)	Saturated Fat (gm)	Trans Fat (gm)	Cholesterol (mg)	Dietary Fiber (gm)	Sodium (mg)	Carbohydrate (gm)	Protein (gm)

Starbucks Coffee ® www.starbucks.com

Product	Total Calories	Total Calories from Fat	Total Fat (gm)	Saturated Fat (gm)	Trans Fat (gm)	Cholesterol (mg)	Dietary Fiber (gm)	Sodium (mg)	Carbohydrate (gm)	Protein (gm)
Caramel	15	0	.5	0	0	0	0	5	2	0
Chocolate Topping	5	0	0	0	0	0	0	0	1	0
Flavored Sugar-free Syrup	0	0	0	0	0	0	0	0	0	0
Mocha Syrup (1 pump)	25	0	.5	0	0	0	0	0	6	1
Flavored Syrup (1 pump)	20	0	0	0	0	0	0	0	5	0
Solo Espresso	5	0	0	0	0	0	0	0	1	0
Tall Brewed Coffee	5	0	0	0	0	0	0	10	1	0
Tall Brewed Tazo Tea	0	0	0	0	0	0	0	0	0	0
Tall Caffe Americano	10	0	0	0	0	0	0	0	2	1
Tall Caramel Frappuccino® Light Blended Coffee	130	10	1	0	0	5	2	180	2	4
Tall Coffee Frappuccino® Light Blended Coffee	90	5	.5	0	0	0	2	160	18	4
Tall Iced Caffe Americano	10	0	0	0	0	0	0	0	2	0
Tall Iced Coffee (with sugar-free syrup)	10	0	0	0	0	0	0	0	0	1
Tall Nonfat Caffe Latte	100	0	0	0	0	5	0	120	15	10
Tall Nonfat Caffe Mocha (no whipped cream)	170	15	1.5	0	0	<5	1	135	33	11
Tall Nonfat Cappuccino	60	0	0	0	0	<5	0	70	9	6

Starbucks Coffee ® (cont.)

Product	Total Calories	Total Calories from Fat	Total Fat (gm)	Saturated Fat (gm)	Trans Fat (gm)	Cholesterol (mg)	Dietary Fiber (gm)	Sodium (mg)	Carbohydrate (gm)	Protein (gm)
Tall Nonfat Caramel Macchiato	140	10	1	.5	0	5	0	105	25	8
Tall Nonfat Iced Caffe Latte	70	0	0	0	0	<5	1	80	10	6
Tall Nonfat Iced Caramel Macchiato	140	5	1	.5	0	5	0	120	25	8
Tall Nonfat Iced Tazo® Chai Black Tea Latte	130	0	0	0	0	5	0	75	26	6
Tall Nonfat Iced Vanilla Latte	120	0	0	0	0	0	0	90	24	6
Tall Nonfat Tazo® Green Tea Latte	160	0	0	0	0	5	1	85	32	7
Tall Caffé Vanilla Frappuccino® Light Blended Coffee	140	5	.5	0	0	2	0	180	30	4
Tall Shaken Tazo® Iced Black Tea Lemonade	100	0	0	0	0	0	0	10	25	0
Tall Shaken Tazo® Iced Passion™ Tea	60	0	0	0	0	0	0	10	16	0
Tall Soy Tazo® Chai Tea Latte	170	20	2	0	0	0	1	65	35	4
Tall Steamed Apple Juice	170	0	0	0	0	0	0	15	43	0
Tall Vanilla Crème (nonfat)	220	60	6	0	0	30	0	125	30	10
Whipped Cream (on tall cold beverages)	80	70	8	5	0	30	0	10	2	0

Product	Total Calories	Total Calories from Fat	Total Fat (gm)	Saturated Fat (gm)	Trans Fat (gm)	Cholesterol (mg)	Dietary Fiber (gm)	Sodium (mg)	Carbohydrate (gm)	Protein (gm)
Subway ®								*www.subway.com*		
4" Mini Ham Sandwich	180	25	3	1	0	10	3	710	30	11
4" Mini Roast Beef Sandwich	190	30	3.5	1.5	0	15	3	600	30	13
4" Mini Turkey Breast Sandwich	190	25	3	1	0	15	3	670	30	12
6" Jared Ham Sandwich	290	45	5	1.5	0	25	4	1260	47	18
6" Jared Oven Roasted Sandwich	310	50	5	1.5	0	25	5	830	4	24
6" Jared Roast Beef Sandwich	290	45	5	2	0	20	4	900	45	19
6" Jared Subway® Club	320	50	6	2	0	35	4	1290	47	24
6" Jared Sweet Onion Chicken Teriyaki Sandwich	370	45	5	1.5	0	50	5	1200	59	26
6" Jared Turkey Breast Sandwich	280	40	4.5	1.5	0	20	4	1000	46	18
6" Jared Turkey Breast and Ham Sandwich	290	45	5	1.5	0	25	4	1210	47	20
6" Jared Veggie Delite®	230	30	3	1	0	0	4	500	44	9
Chicken and Dumpling Soup	170	45	5	2	0	35	2	1390	23	8
Chili Con Carne	290	70	8	3.5	0	25	12	990	35	19
Fat-Free Italian Dressing	35	0	0	0	0	0	0	720	7	1

Subway® (cont.)

Product	Total Calories	Total Calories from Fat	Total Fat (gm)	Saturated Fat (gm)	Trans Fat (gm)	Cholesterol (mg)	Dietary Fiber (gm)	Sodium (mg)	Carbohydrate (gm)	Protein (gm)
Jared Ham Salad	120	25	3	1	0	25	4	840	14	12
Jared Oven Roasted Chicken Breast Salad	140	25	2.5	.5	0	50	4	390	11	19
Jared Roast Beef Salad	120	30	3	1.5	0	20	4	480	12	13
Jared Subway® Club Salad	150	35	4	1.5	0	35	4	870	14	18
Jared Sweet Onion Chicken Teriyaki	210	30	3	1	0	50	4	780	26	20
Jared Turkey Breast Salad	110	20	2.5	.5	0	20	4	580	13	12
Jared Veggie Delite®	60	10	1	0	0	0	4	80	11	3
Minestrone	80	10	1	.5	0	<5	4	1125	15	4
Roasted Chicken Noodle Soup	80	20	2	.5	0	15	1	1240	11	6
Spanish Style Chicken with Rice Soup	110	20	2	.5	0	10	1	1300	17	6
Tomato Garden Vegetable Soup with Rotini	90	0	0	0	0	0	2	1140	20	3
Vegetable Beef Soup	100	20	2	.5	0	10	3	1450	15	6

Product	Total Calories	Total Calories from Fat	Total Fat (gm)	Saturated Fat (gm)	Trans Fat (gm)	Cholesterol (mg)	Dietary Fiber (gm)	Sodium (mg)	Carbohydrate (gm)	Protein (gm)

Taco Bell ®

www.tacobell.com

Product	Total Calories	Total Calories from Fat	Total Fat (gm)	Saturated Fat (gm)	Trans Fat (gm)	Cholesterol (mg)	Dietary Fiber (gm)	Sodium (mg)	Carbohydrate (gm)	Protein (gm)
1/2 lb. Cheesy Bean and Rice Burrito	330	70	7	2	0	0	6	1080	55	10
7-Layer Burrito	380	80	8	2.5	.5	0	9	1190	62	13
Bean Burrito	350	81	9	3.5	.5	5	8	1190	54	13
Chili Cheese Burrito	270	70	8	3	0	15	4	930	39	10
Crunchy Taco	150	70	8	2.5	0	20	3	370	13	7
Crunchy Taco Supreme®	170	90	10	3.5	0	25	3	350	14	8
Enchiritos® (beef)	230	80	8	3.5	.5	20	7	1300	34	12
Fiesta Burrito (beef)	350	99	11	4	0	20	5	1220	49	12
Fiesta Burrito (chicken)	350	90	10	3.5	0	30	3	1220	47	18
Grilled Steak Soft Taco	160	40	4.5	1.5	0	20	2	550	20	10
Mexican Rice	110	25	3	0	0	0	1	460	19	2
MexiMelt®	190	70	7	3	0	20	3	710	22	8
Pintos 'n Cheese	120	20	2	0	.5	0	7	640	19	6
Ranchero Chicken Soft Taco	170	35	4	1.5	0	25	3	730	21	12
Soft Taco (beef)	180	70	7	3	0	20	3	860	21	8
Soft Taco Supreme® (beef)	190	70	7	3	0	20	3	650	22	9
Spicy Chicken Soft Taco	170	50	6	2	0	25	2	649	22	10
Steak Grilled Taquitos	260	60	7	2.5	0	20	3	830	37	13
Tostado	200	54	6	1	.5	0	8	700	27	7

Taco John's®

www.tacojohns.com

Product	Total Calories	Total Calories from Fat	Total Fat (gm)	Saturated Fat (gm)	Trans Fat (gm)	Cholesterol (mg)	Dietary Fiber (gm)	Sodium (mg)	Carbohydrate (gm)	Protein (gm)
Bean Burrito (without cheese)	320	60	7	2	2	<5	10	740	53	11
Chicken Soft Taco	190	50	6	3	1	30	4	760	19	14
Crispy Taco	180	90	10	4	0	25	3	270	13	9
Giant Goldfish Grahams	120	35	5	1	0	<5	1	110	19	1
Mexi Rolls® (2 pc. without cheese)	155	65	7	2	0	15	6	195	16	8
Mexican Rice	240	70	8	2	1	<5	1	1100	36	4
Pico de Gallo (1 oz.)	5	0	0	0	0	<5	0	85	2	0
Refried Beans (without cheese)	340	80	9	3	4	<5	11	1030	49	15
Salsa (1 oz.)	20	0	0	0	0	<5	1	220	4	1
Side Salad (without dressing)	80	40	5	0	0	5	1	50	6	3
Soft Taco	230	94	10	5	0	25	3	590	20	11
Taco Burger (without cheese)	250	90	9	3	0	25	3	560	30	13
Texas Style Chili (without cheese)	210	70	8	3	1	20	4	1310	26	11

Product	Total Calories	Total Calories from Fat	Total Fat (gm)	Saturated Fat (gm)	Trans Fat (gm)	Cholesterol (mg)	Dietary Fiber (gm)	Sodium (mg)	Carbohydrate (gm)	Protein (gm)

Wendy's ®

www.wendys.com

Product	Total Calories	Total Calories from Fat	Total Fat (gm)	Saturated Fat (gm)	Trans Fat (gm)	Cholesterol (mg)	Dietary Fiber (gm)	Sodium (mg)	Carbohydrate (gm)	Protein (gm)
Chicken Caesar Salad (without dressing)	180	60	6	2.5	0	70	3	660	8	25
Crispy Noodles	60	20	2	0	0	0	0	170	10	1
Fat-Free French Dressing	70	0	0	0	0	0	0	190	17	0
Homestyle Chicken Fillet sandwich	430	160	16	2.5	0	45	2	1140	48	25
Homestyle Garlic Croutons	70	25	2.5	0	0	0	0	125	9	2
Hot Chili Seasoning	5	0	0	0	0	0	0	270	2	0
Jr. Hamburger	230	70	8	3	0	30	1	490	27	13
Junior Frosty™ (chocolate)	160	35	4	2.5	0	15	0	75	26	4
Junior Frosty™ (vanilla)	150	35	4	2.5	0	20	0	90	26	4
Low-Fat Honey Mustard	100	25	2.5	0	0	0	0	300	19	0
Low-Fat Strawberry Flavored Yogurt	140	15	1.5	1	0	5	0	90	27	6
Mandarin Chicken® Salad	170	25	2.5	.5	0	60	3	520	16	21
Mandarin Orange Cup	80	0	0	0	0	0	1	15	19	1
Plain Baked Potato	270	0	0	0	0	0	7	25	61	7
Roasted Almonds	130	110	11	1	0	0	2	70	4	5
Saltine Crackers	25	5	.5	0	0	0	0	95	4	0
Side Salad	35	0	0	0	0	0	2	25	8	1

Product	Total Calories	Total Calories from Fat	Total Fat (gm)	Saturated Fat (gm)	Trans Fat (gm)	Cholesterol (mg)	Dietary Fiber (gm)	Sodium (mg)	Carbohydrate (gm)	Protein (gm)

Wendy's® (cont.)

Product	Total Calories	Total Calories from Fat	Total Fat (gm)	Saturated Fat (gm)	Trans Fat (gm)	Cholesterol (mg)	Dietary Fiber (gm)	Sodium (mg)	Carbohydrate (gm)	Protein (gm)
Small Chili	220	60	6	2.5	0	35	5	780	23	17
Spicy Chicken Sandwich	440	160	16	2.5	0	60	3	1320	46	28
Ultimate Chicken Grill Sandwich	320	70	7	1.5	0	70	2	950	3	28

Whataburger®   www.whataburger.com

Product	Total Calories	Total Calories from Fat	Total Fat (gm)	Saturated Fat (gm)	Trans Fat (gm)	Cholesterol (mg)	Dietary Fiber (gm)	Sodium (mg)	Carbohydrate (gm)	Protein (gm)
Whataburger Jr.®	320	140	16	5	.5	30	1	861	32	14

For more information about
First Place 4 Health,
please contact:

First Place 4 Health
7025 West Tidwell, Suite H101
Houston, TX 77092
1-800-72-PLACE (727-5223)
email: info@firstplace4health.com
website: www.firstplace4health.com